Adventures
on the
Can Do Trail

By Jothy Rosenberg
Illustrations by Mary Garica

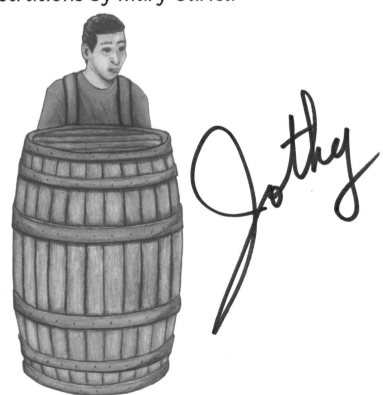

Copyright © 2022 by **Jothy Rosenberg**
Illustrations Copyright © 2022 by **Mary Garcia**

Library of Congress Control Number: 2022917480

ISBN 979-8-218-07559-0 (hardback)
ISBN 979-8-88759-139-1 (paperback)
ISBN 979-8-88759-140-7 (ebook)

First hardback edition October 2022
Wayland, Massachusetts

$1 from each book sold goes to the Who Says I Can't Foundation (whosaysicant.org)

Book design by Jothy Rosenberg

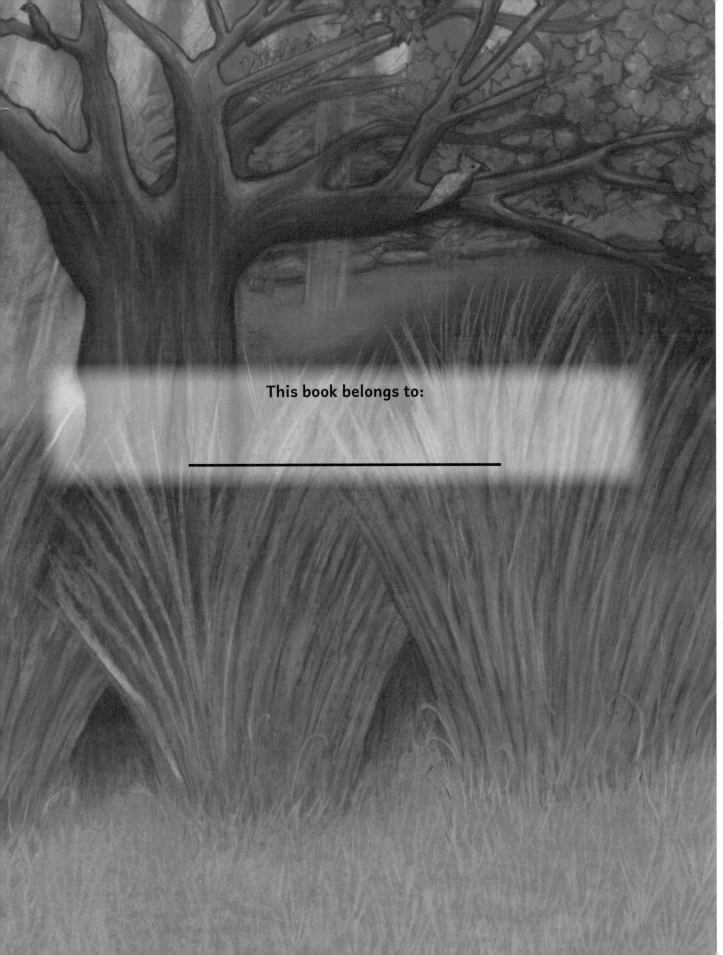

This book belongs to:

_____

Note to readers

When you or your readees encounter the word

CAN'T say it with sadness.

But, when you encounter the phrase

WHO SAYS I CAN'T (in all caps) it is not a

question, it is a statement and please shout out the word

SAYS with glee to make the point!

Dedications

Jothy's:
to Bowen, Warner, and Bram, grandsons at just the perfect age for this book.

Mary's:
the illustrations in this book are dedicated to all those like me with invisible disabilities.

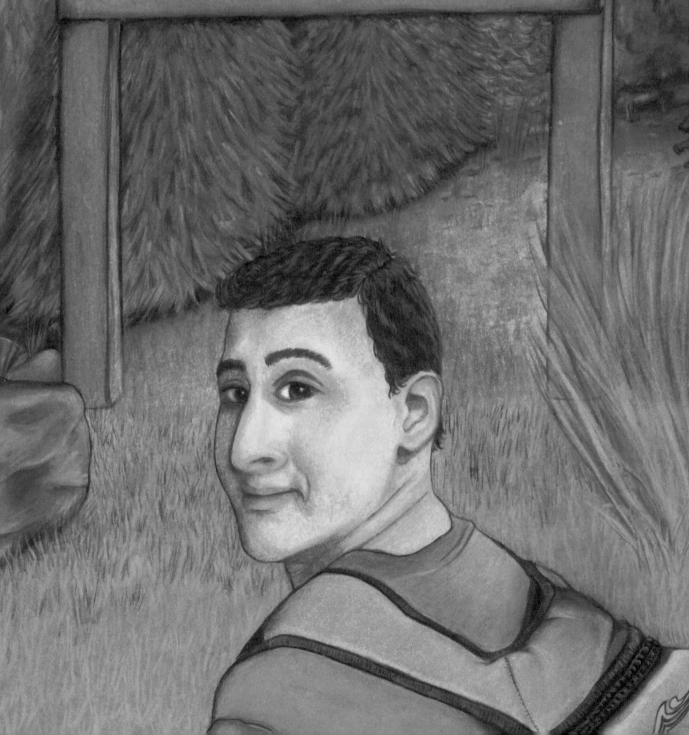

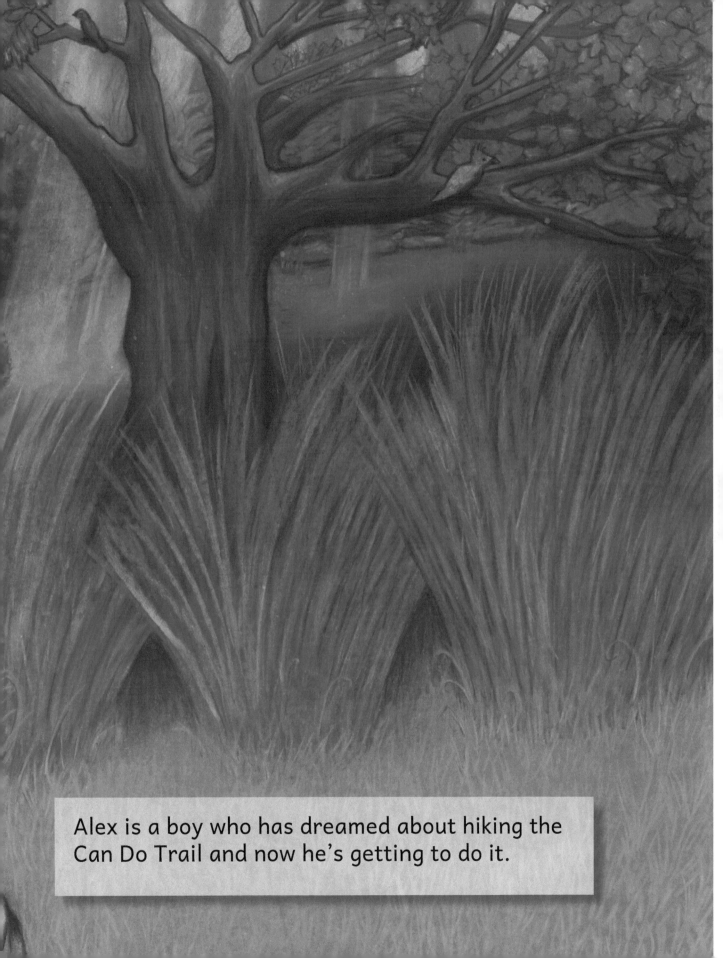

Alex is a boy who has dreamed about hiking the Can Do Trail and now he's getting to do it.

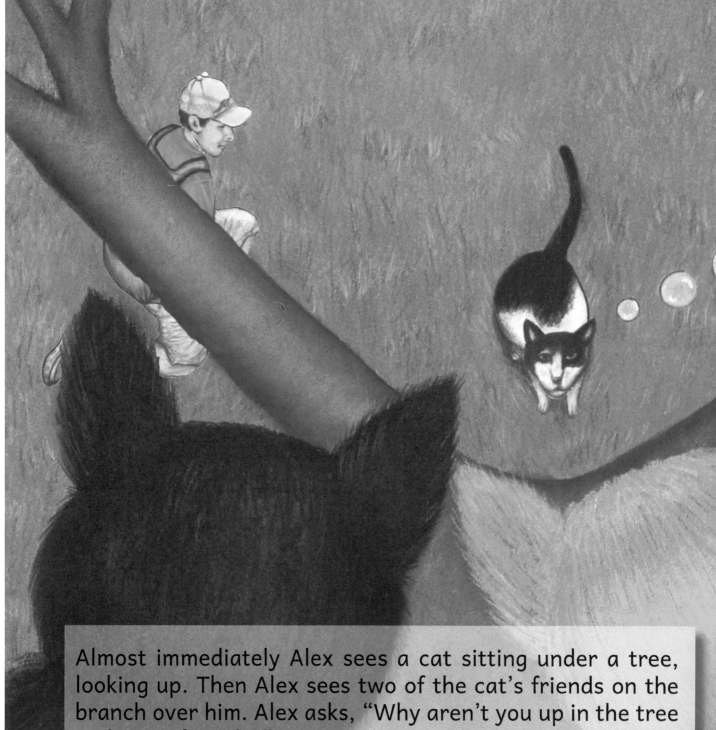

Almost immediately Alex sees a cat sitting under a tree, looking up. Then Alex sees two of the cat's friends on the branch over him. Alex asks, "Why aren't you up in the tree with your friends?"

The cat softly says, "I have no claws, so **I CAN'T** climb trees. It makes me sad because I want to be with my friends."

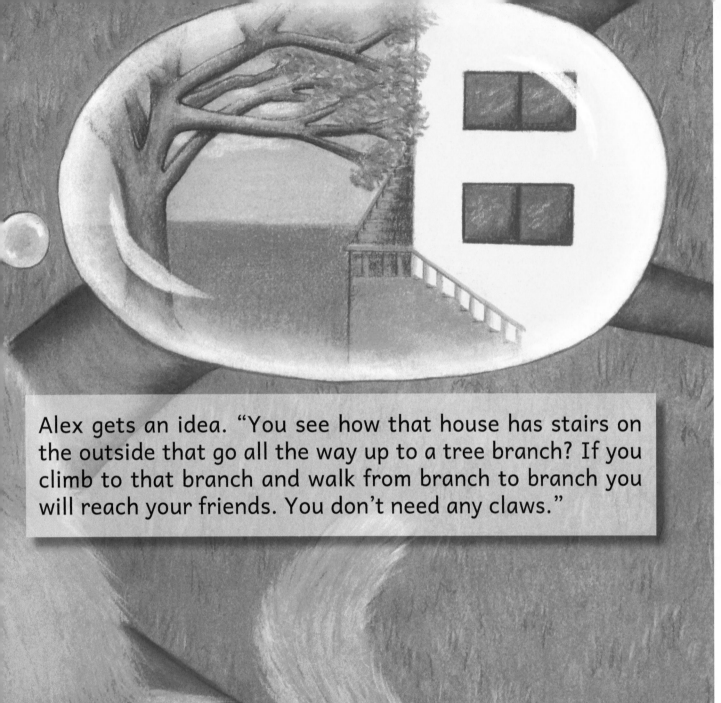

Alex gets an idea. "You see how that house has stairs on the outside that go all the way up to a tree branch? If you climb to that branch and walk from branch to branch you will reach your friends. You don't need any claws."

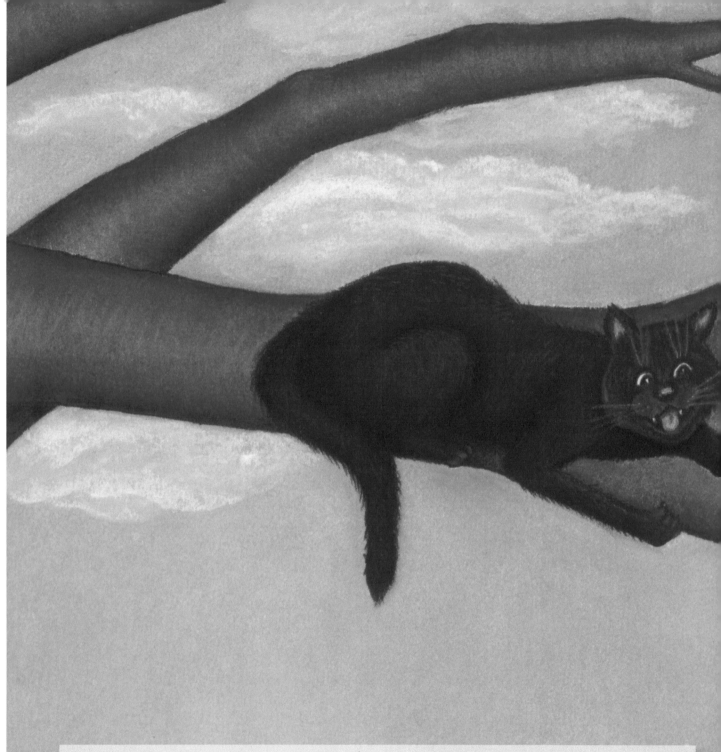

The cat runs happily up the stairs. She joins her friends in the tree and they give each other high fives. The cat with no claws looks down and purrs to Alex, "I am the cat with no claws, but **WHO SAYS I CAN'T** climb trees!"

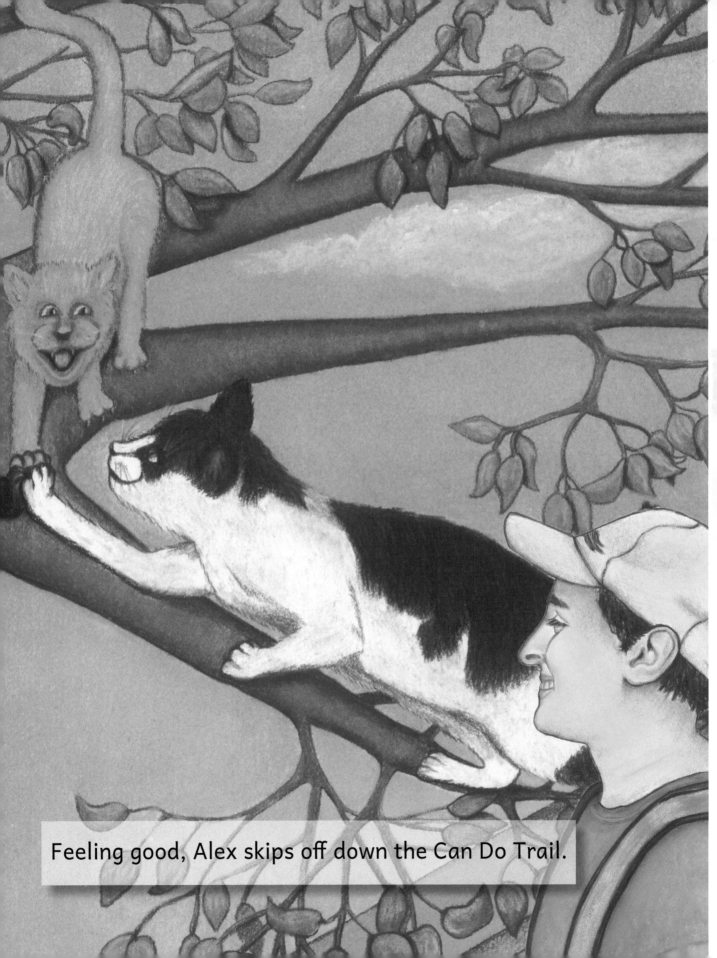

Feeling good, Alex skips off down the Can Do Trail.

Alex arrives next in the Wet Lands, where he sees two herons talking. Much to Alex's surprise, one has no feathers. Alex asks her if she can fly.

The other heron answers, "No, a bird without feathers **CAN'T** fly. So, my cousin will not be able to fly south with us when the cold weather comes. I am worried she will freeze."

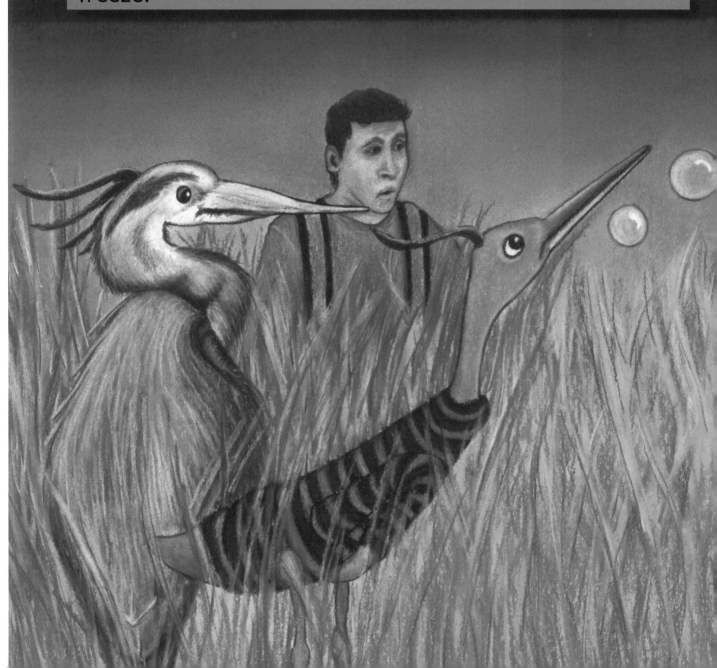

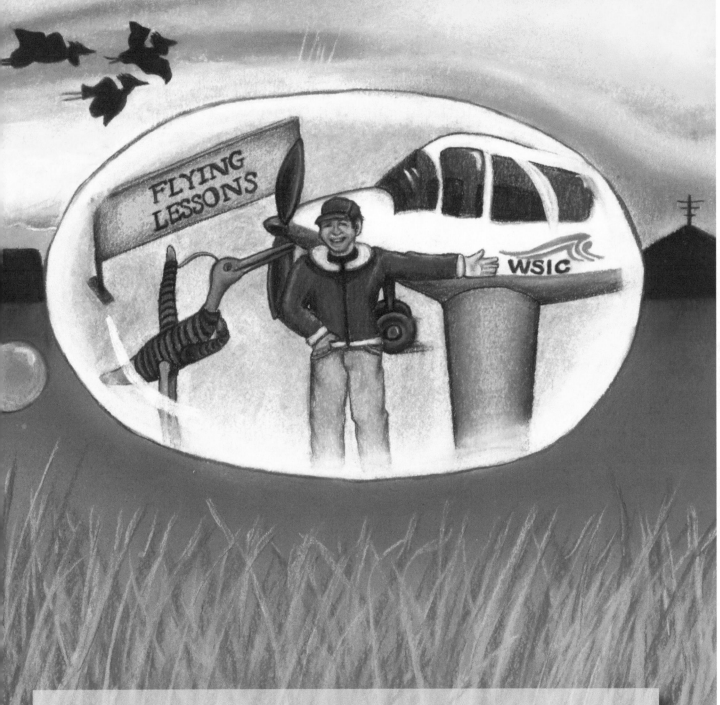

Alex notices a sign at the airport nearby advertising flying lessons, and he gets an idea. Alex talks to the teacher who agrees to teach the heron with no feathers how to fly a plane. The heron adapts easily to flying a plane. She and her cousin are very relieved and happy that she can now fly.

A flock of herons flies alongside the plane as it flies low in the sky. Through the plane's window, the bird says, "I am the heron with no feathers, but **WHO SAYS I CAN'T** fly!" And with that, the entire flock heads south for a warm winter.

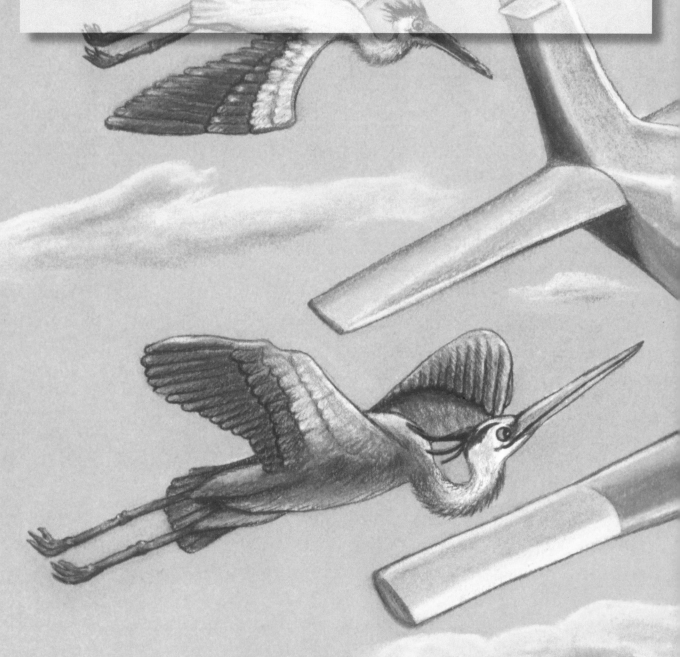

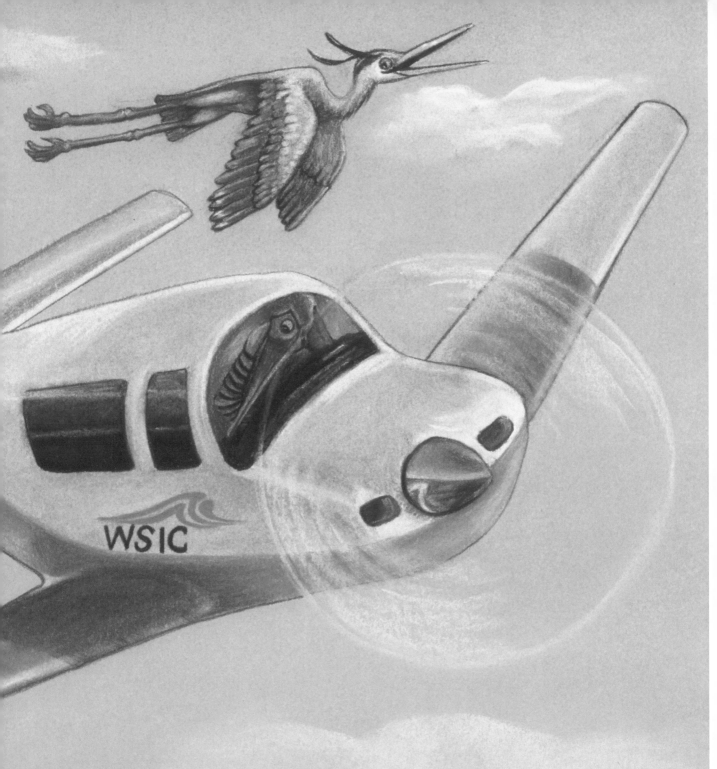

Alex heads on down the Can Do Trail, thrilled for his next adventure.

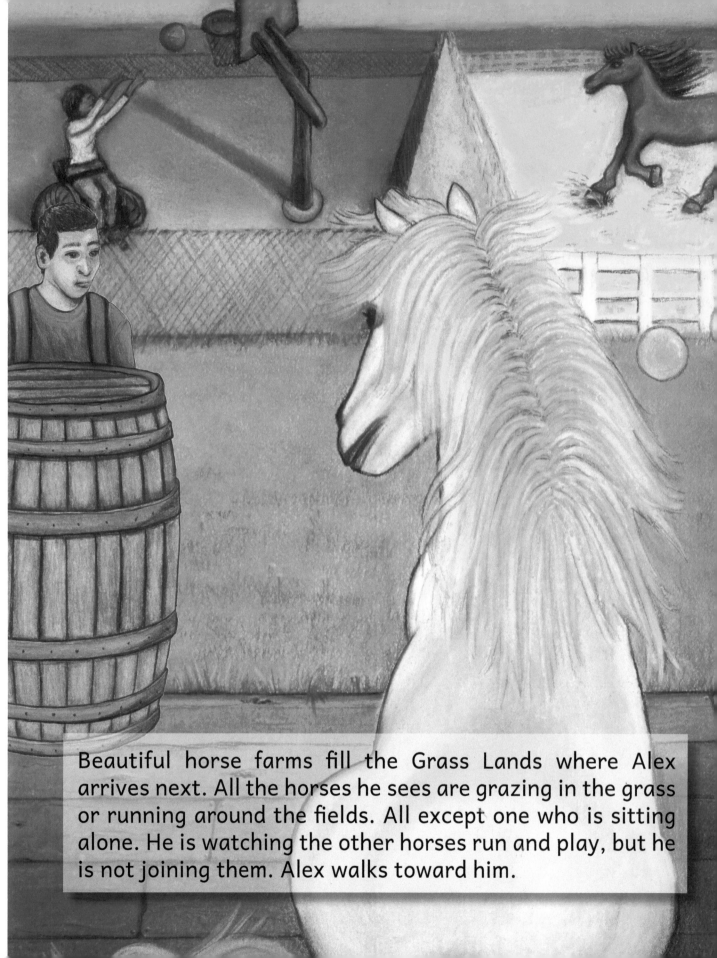

Beautiful horse farms fill the Grass Lands where Alex arrives next. All the horses he sees are grazing in the grass or running around the fields. All except one who is sitting alone. He is watching the other horses run and play, but he is not joining them. Alex walks toward him.

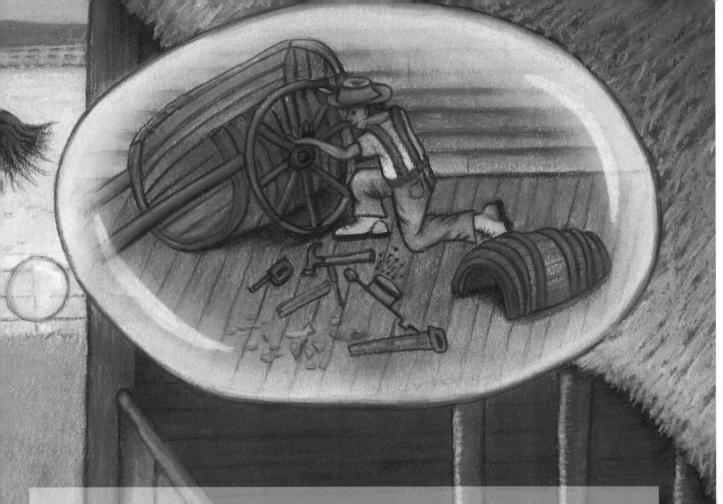

Alex realizes this horse has no back legs and is clearly sad to be by himself.

"Horses are meant to run," the little horse says to Alex. "I'm always left behind and stared at because I don't have back legs. My friends say I **CAN'T** run and chase them like a horse should."

Just then, Alex sees a child in a wheelchair playing basketball and gets an idea. The farmer loves Alex's idea because he loves his horse and wants to help him. Alex and the farmer work together to create a beautiful half-wheelchair, half-chariot and they fit it to the horse.

With a little practice, the horse is walking, then running. He can catch his friends now! He is so happy he can't stop whinnying.

"Neigh! Neigh! I am the horse with no back legs, but **WHO SAYS I CAN'T** run!"

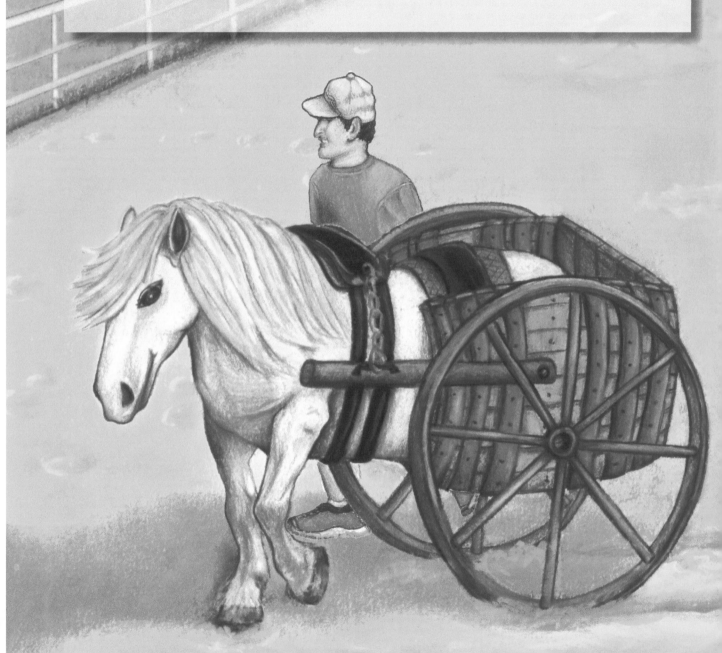

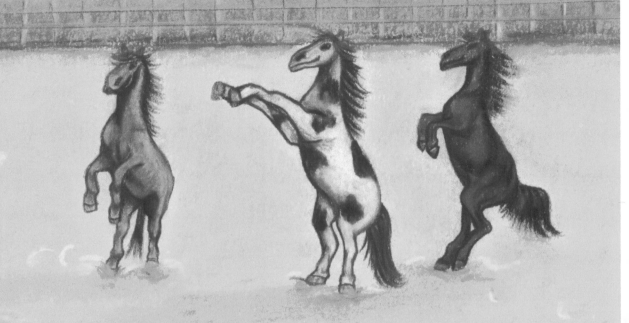

He paws with his front legs and takes off for the back of the field, where his friends are waiting for him. The farmer is happy too.

Alex says good-bye and heads on down the Can Do Trail.

Next up are the Sea Coast Lands where Alex comes upon an animal hospital where sick or injured sea mammals are cared for in large pools. In one pool is a dolphin who has no tail.

Alex knows a dolphin uses its powerful tail to propel itself through the water. "How do you swim?" He asks.

The dolphin says, "Without my tail flukes, **I CAN'T** swim. **I CAN'T** catch fish. **I CAN'T** be with my pod. I will have to stay here in this pen for my whole life and have the humans feed me fish." Using just his front fins, he slowly moves to the other side of the pool.

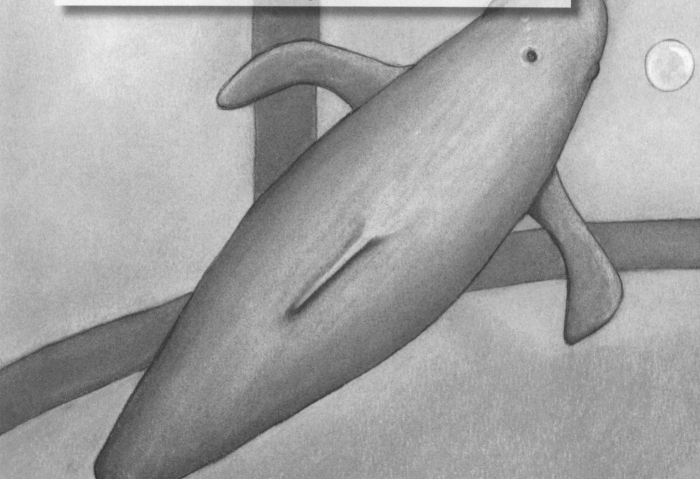

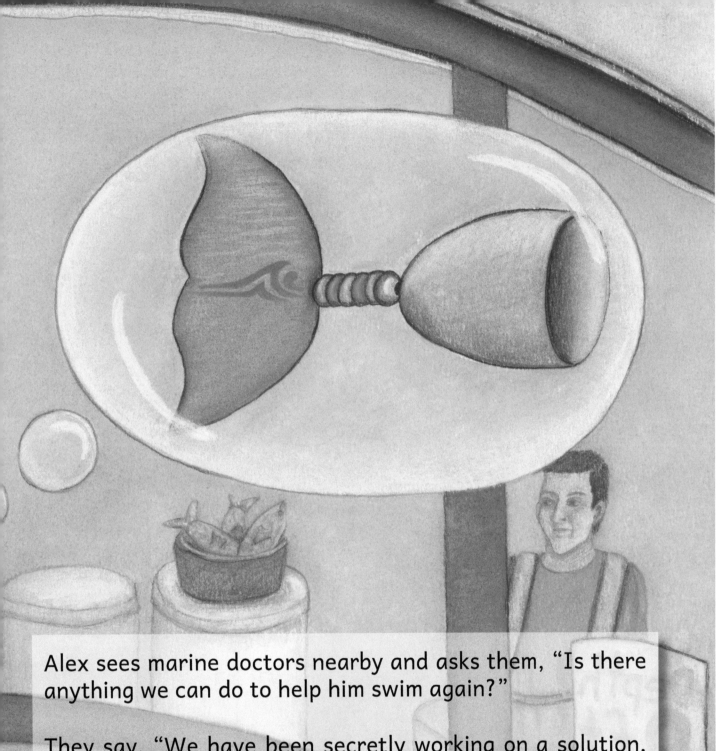

Alex sees marine doctors nearby and asks them, "Is there anything we can do to help him swim again?"

They say, "We have been secretly working on a solution, but we did not want to get the dolphin's hopes up."

They have made a special plastic tail and flukes. They ask if Alex will help them attach it.

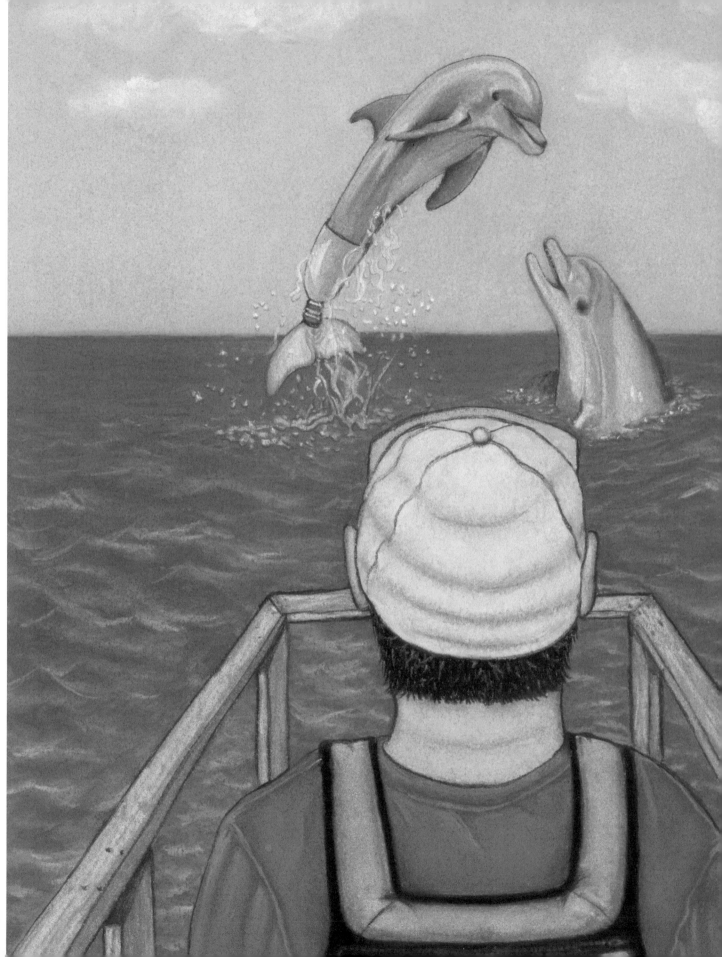

They carefully fit the man-made tail, called a "prosthesis," onto the dolphin. With this special prosthesis, the dolphin can zoom around the pen and even leap out of the water.

He makes clicks and screeches with delight saying, "I am the dolphin with no tail flukes but **WHO SAYS I CAN'T** swim and jump!"

Alex opens the dolphin's pen door, and the dolphin joyfully splashes out into the open ocean to join his pod and catch his own fish.

Alex is very proud as he travels inland on the Can Do Trail.

Many creatures, large and small, make their home in the Forest Lands. Alex happens upon a pair of owls talking.

One of them says, "I am the owl with no night vision. I **CAN'T** hunt at night when all the delicious little rodents are out. How will I get enough to eat?"

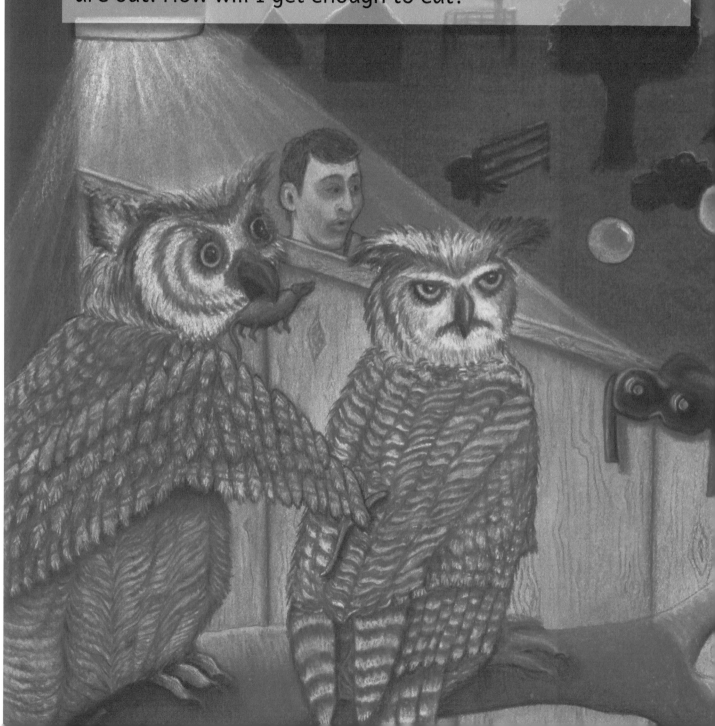

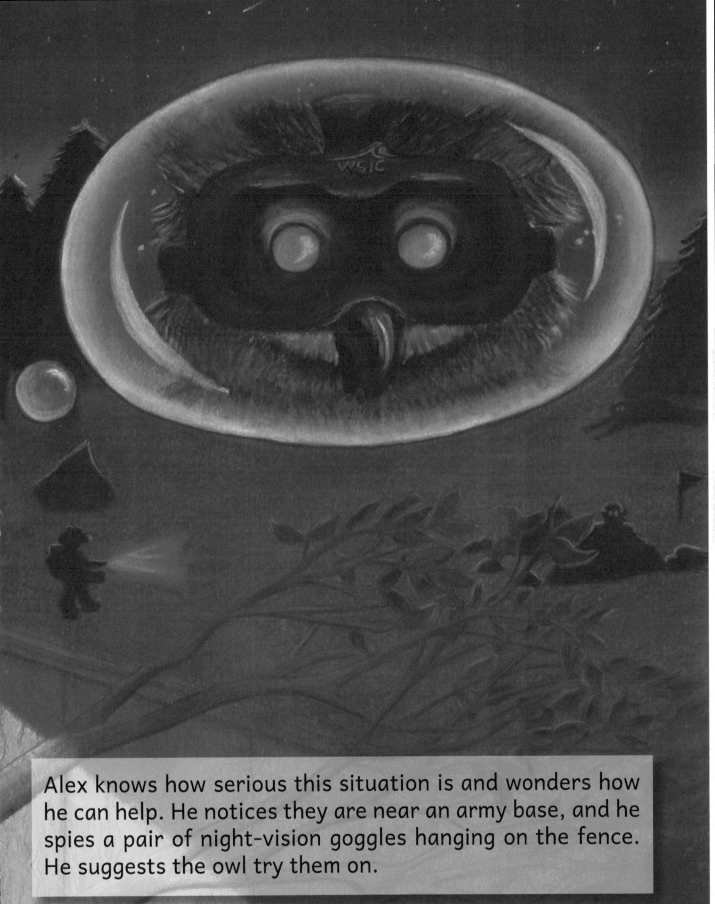

Alex knows how serious this situation is and wonders how he can help. He notices they are near an army base, and he spies a pair of night-vision goggles hanging on the fence. He suggests the owl try them on.

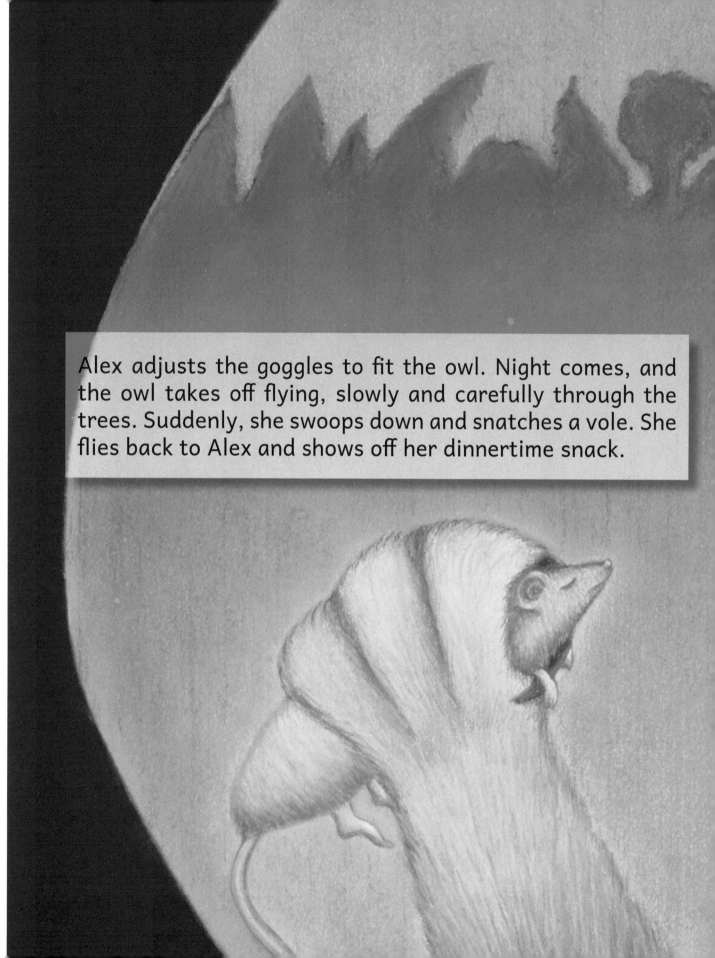

Alex adjusts the goggles to fit the owl. Night comes, and the owl takes off flying, slowly and carefully through the trees. Suddenly, she swoops down and snatches a vole. She flies back to Alex and shows off her dinnertime snack.

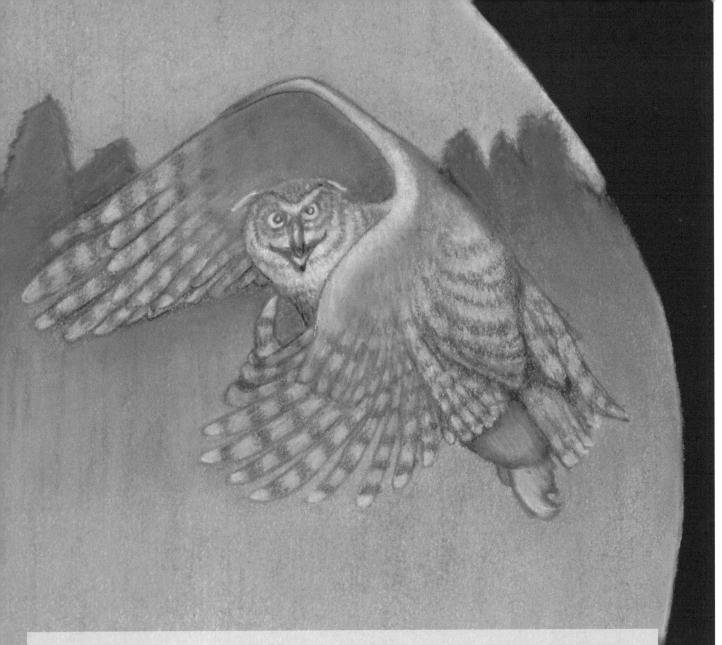

"I am the owl with no night vision but **WHO SAYS I CAN'T** fly and hunt at night!" she says as she gobbles down her dinner. She joyfully cries out, "Hoot! Hoot!" and silently soars away to go find more food deeper in the dark forest.

Alex proudly watches the owl fly away and then heads down the Can Do Trail.

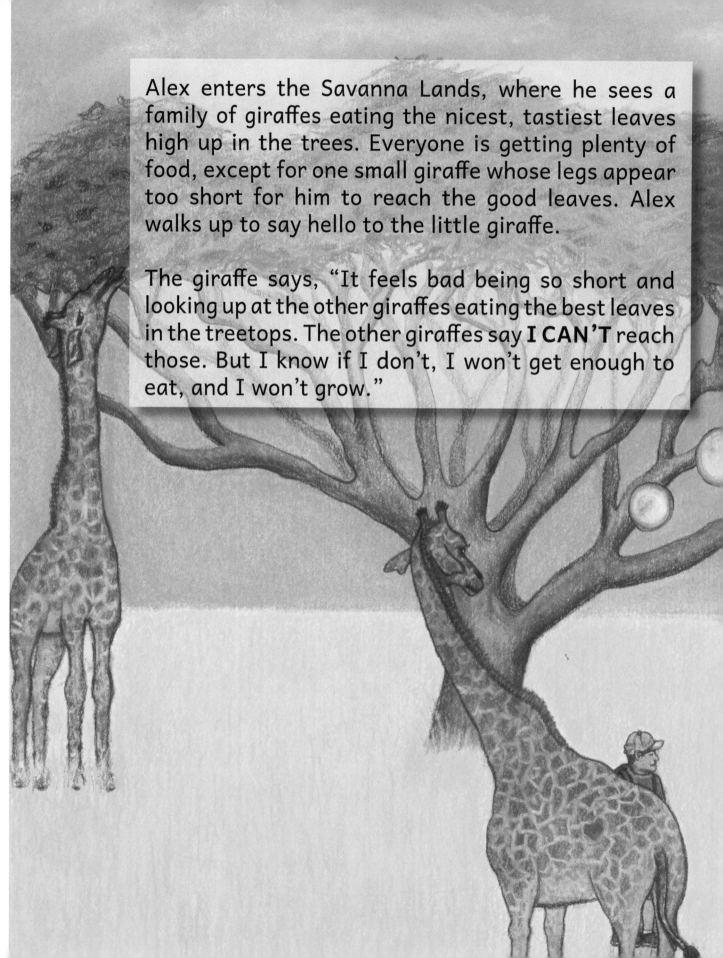

Alex enters the Savanna Lands, where he sees a family of giraffes eating the nicest, tastiest leaves high up in the trees. Everyone is getting plenty of food, except for one small giraffe whose legs appear too short for him to reach the good leaves. Alex walks up to say hello to the little giraffe.

The giraffe says, "It feels bad being so short and looking up at the other giraffes eating the best leaves in the treetops. The other giraffes say **I CAN'T** reach those. But I know if I don't, I won't get enough to eat, and I won't grow."

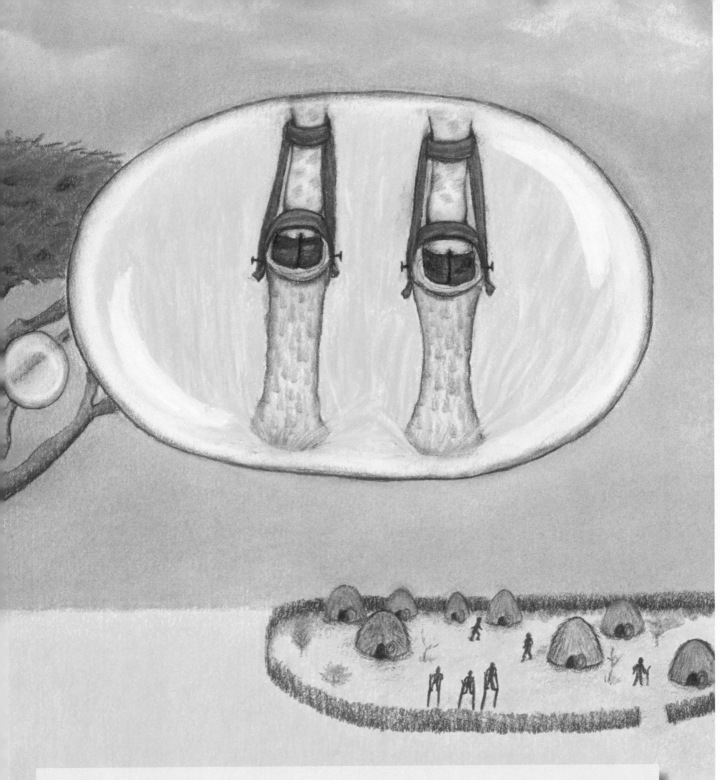

Nearby, Alex sees a human village, where several of the children are having fun standing very tall on stilts giving Alex an idea.

When Alex comes back, he has a set of stilts he helps the giraffe strap on. With some practice, the giraffe can walk well. Now the little giraffe is not so little. In fact, he's taller than his father! He's able to eat leaves that even his father cannot.

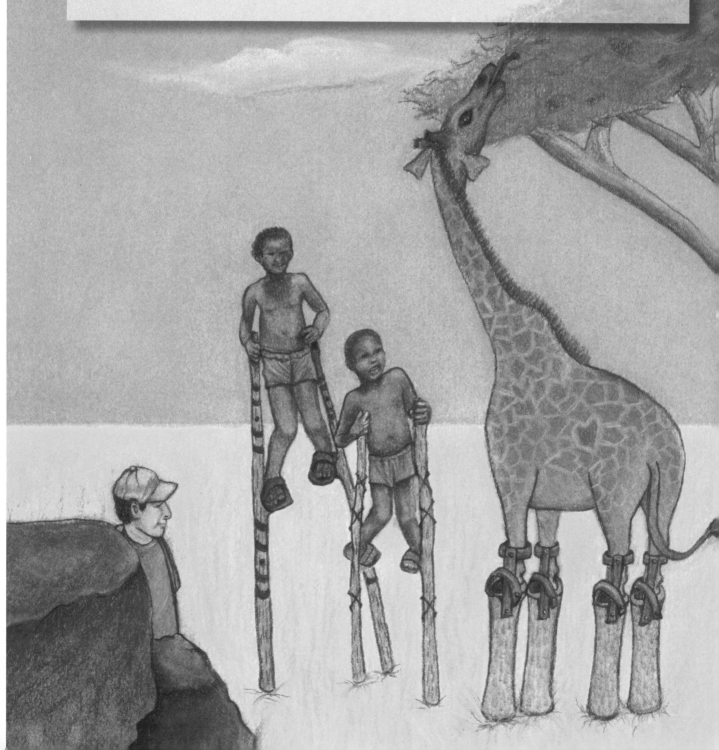

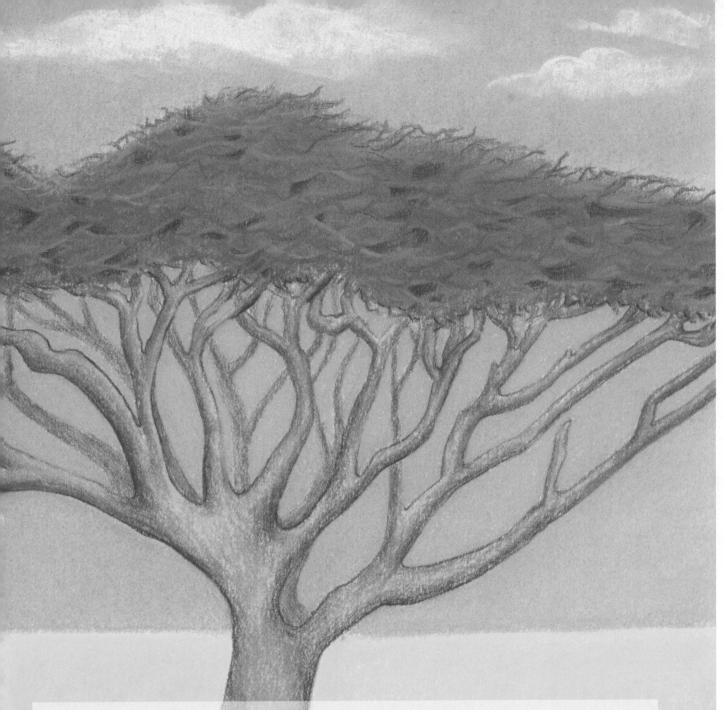

"Woo-hoo!" he says. "I am the giraffe with short legs, but **WHO SAYS I CAN'T** make myself tall and reach the best leaves at the treetops!"

Feeling satisfied, Alex leaves the giraffes for the last stop on the Can Do Trail.

Entering the High Lands, Alex is hoping to see the most impressive resident living there: the wolf. Wolves are elusive, but eventually he finds a wolf pack. They are hunting, always talking with each other as they work as a unit. However, one is sitting on a rock, just watching.

Alex goes over to her and asks, "Why are you not part of the hunting group?"

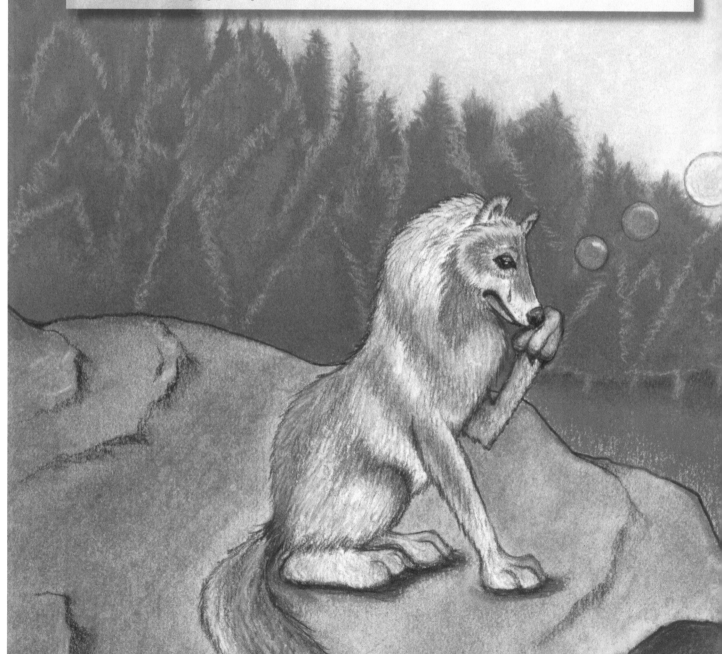

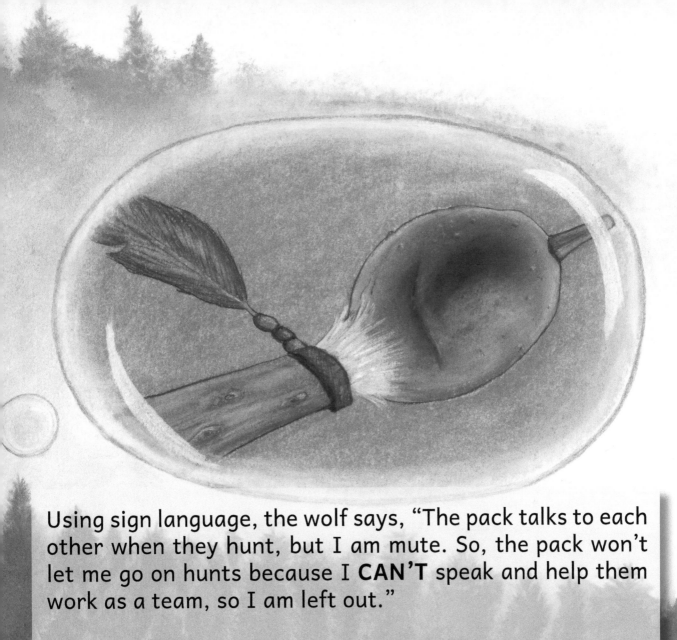

Using sign language, the wolf says, "The pack talks to each other when they hunt, but I am mute. So, the pack won't let me go on hunts because I **CAN'T** speak and help them work as a team, so I am left out."

Alex looks thoughtfully at the wolf as he ponders how he can help her overcome her muteness. Suddenly, Alex remembers a musical instrument made from hollow sticks he used to bang together. He searches for the right kind of branches and hollows them out.

Alex shows his creation to the lone wolf and teaches her how to use the sticks to make a loud "click-click" sound that will travel great distances. The wolf tries it and is delighted. She runs off to join the pack. When she needs to tell the pack which way to go during a hunt, she says "click-click" with her new sticks. The other wolves follow her lead and move as a unit. They catch the prey they are chasing, thanks to the mute wolf and her sticks.

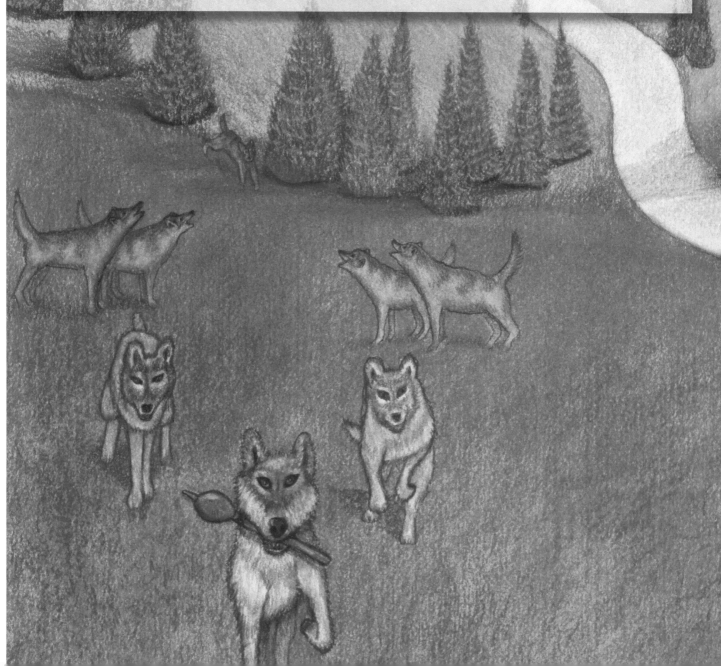

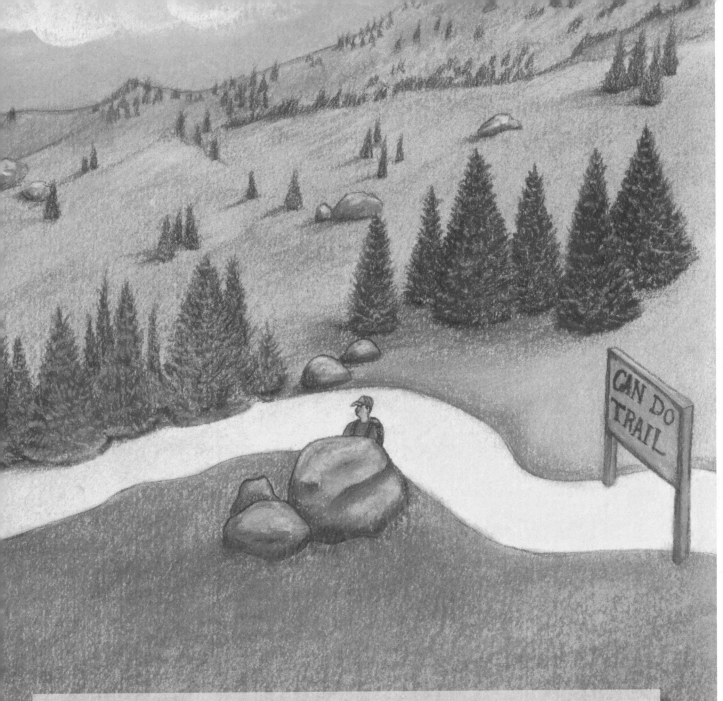

"Click-click!" the mute wolf says with her sticks. To Alex, in sign language, she says, "I am the wolf with no voice, but **WHO SAYS I CAN'T** communicate and help my pack hunt!"

Alex is at the end of the Can Do Trail, and he is so happy he jumps up very high and clicks his heels together.

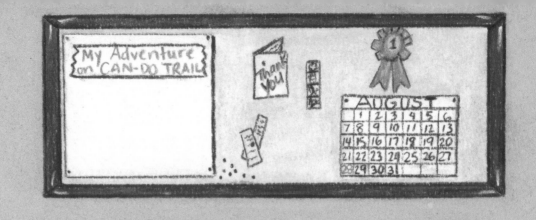

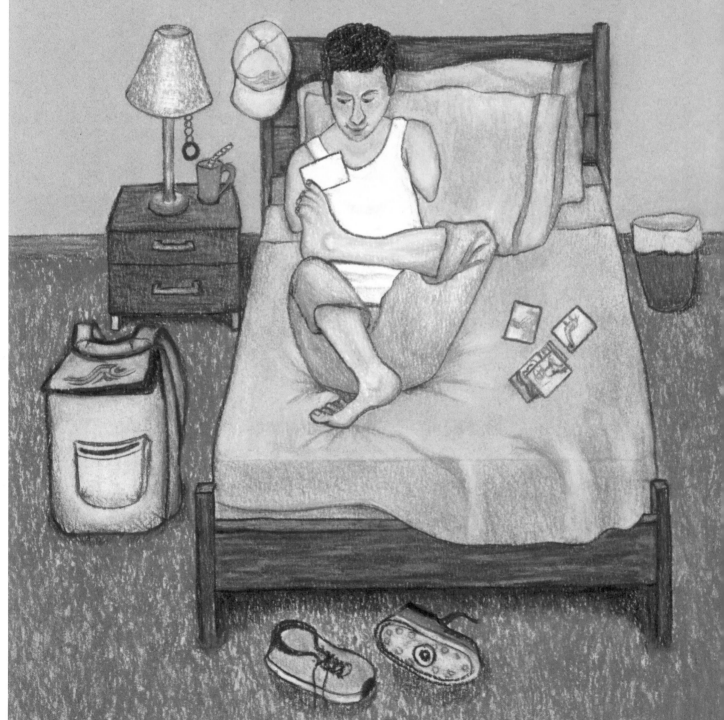

Alex saw amazing things and found ways to help every animal he met facing a challenge to adapt and overcome. Thank goodness he had lots of practice doing things with his feet and his arm stubs.

Alex thinks to himself, "I may be a boy who was born without arms, but **WHO SAYS I CAN'T** do what I want to do in my life! **I CAN** do what I want because I try different ways—and never give up—until I find what works!"

Scavenger Hunt
Can you find these things?

Welcome
- [ ] red bird
- [ ] yellow bird
- [ ] backpack
- [ ] Who Says I Can't logo

Cats
- [ ] cat with no claws
- [ ] Who Says I Can't logo

Heron
- [ ] sweater
- [ ] airport
- [ ] airplane
- [ ] Who Says I Can't logo

Wolf
- [ ] feather
- [ ] wolf tears
- [ ] noise maker
- [ ] wolf howling
- [ ] trail sign
- [ ] Who Says I Can't logo

Dolphin
- [ ] sign says fish basket "depth 8 ft"
- [ ] fish
- [ ] basket
- [ ] railing
- [ ] prosthetic tail
- [ ] Who Says I Can't logo

Horse
- [ ] child in a wheelchair
- [ ] measuring tape
- [ ] barrel
- [ ] basketball net
- [ ] yellow shoes
- [ ] Who Says I Can't logo
- [ ] saw
- [ ] hammer
- [ ] farmer
- [ ] nails
- [ ] drill
- [ ] saddle
- [ ] basketball
- [ ] hat
- [ ] wheel

Giraffe
- [ ] thatch huts
- [ ] villagers
- [ ] stilts
- [ ] Who Says I Can't logo

Owl
- [ ] night vision goggles
- [ ] buildings
- [ ] jeep
- [ ] soldier
- [ ] worm
- [ ] vole
- [ ] Who Says I Can't logo

Alex
- [ ] Who Says I Can't logo
- [ ] camera shoe
- [ ] backpack
- [ ] light
- [ ] pillows
- [ ] trash can
- [ ] photos
- [ ] hat
- [ ] blue ribbon
- [ ] drink
- [ ] calendar
- [ ] night stand

Meet the Author

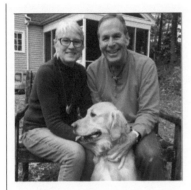

Jothy Rosenberg

Jothy knows a lot about challenge and adversity from losing his leg to bone cancer at age 16. But like Alex and the animals in this book, he conquered and went on to get a PhD in computer science, was a serial entrepreneur starting nine high-tech startups, has authored three technical books, and became an extreme athlete. And like the horse, the heron, and all the others along the Can Do Trail, he was told what he can't do all the time. But he learned to face his challenges and to never say can't and to adapt to and work hard at whatever he wanted to accomplish. Jothy has three young grandsons, Warner, Bowen and Bram, who gave him feedback on this book as it was developing. Jothy loves cookies, pizza, and lasagna. He loves hiking with his dog, swimming, skiing, biking, and visiting with his family and friends. He really loved creating this book and hopes it means kids ban the word CAN'T from their lives.

Jothy lives in Wayland, Massachusetts with his wife Carole and Golden Retriever Harper.

Meet the Illustrator

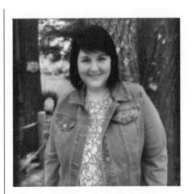

Mary Garcia

Mary Garcia is the author and illustrator of the children's book, "Boo-Boo's New Leg: A True Story of Illness, Acceptance and Healing". She connected with Jothy via social media and accepted the job of illustrating her second book. Things didn't always go as planned though. Mary had to take care of her parents as well as her own children and was also diagnosed with ADD and anxiety. These two invisible disabilities coupled with the life changes she went through proved very tough on Mary, but Jothy was kind, uplifting and patient. Eleven years later she saw through to the end of the project while working as a teacher assistant in a special needs preschool where she is devoted to educating children and using her creative gifts among her school family.

Mary loves her family, pizza with peppers and onions, the color green, jean jackets, cats (she has 4), arts and crafts, music, music and more music, Sharpie markers, praying mantises and her job.

CPSIA information can be obtained
at www.ICGtesting.com
Printed in the USA
BVHW021945221022
649683BV00002B/10